DARWIN DRAGONFLY LEARNS THE SECRET TO *Mindfulness*

WRITTEN BY

TINA R. PARSONS

ILLUSTRATED BY

JENNIFER STABLES

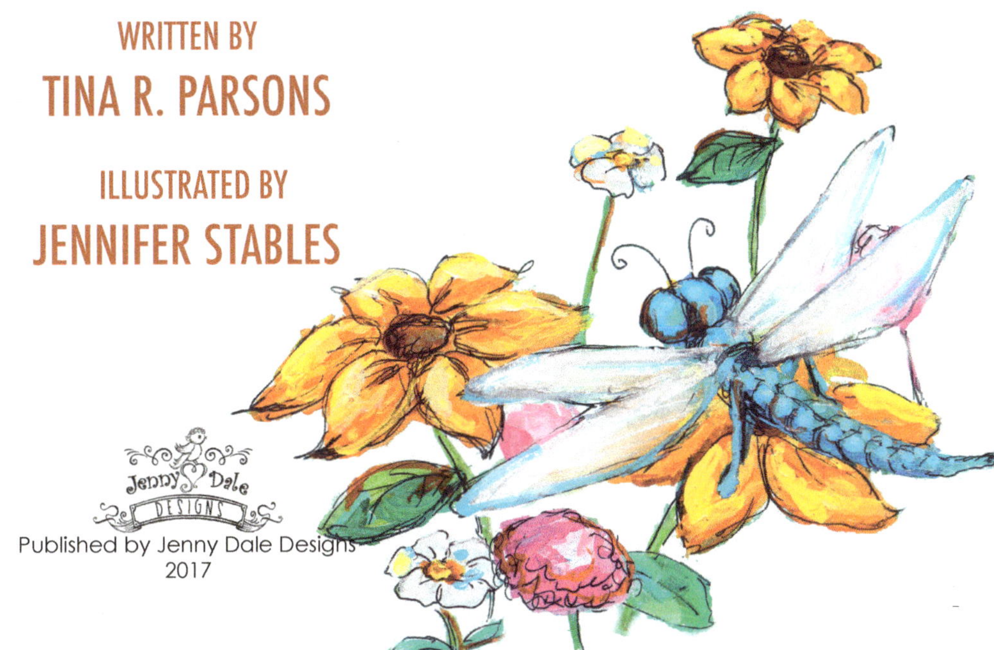

Published by Jenny Dale Designs

2017

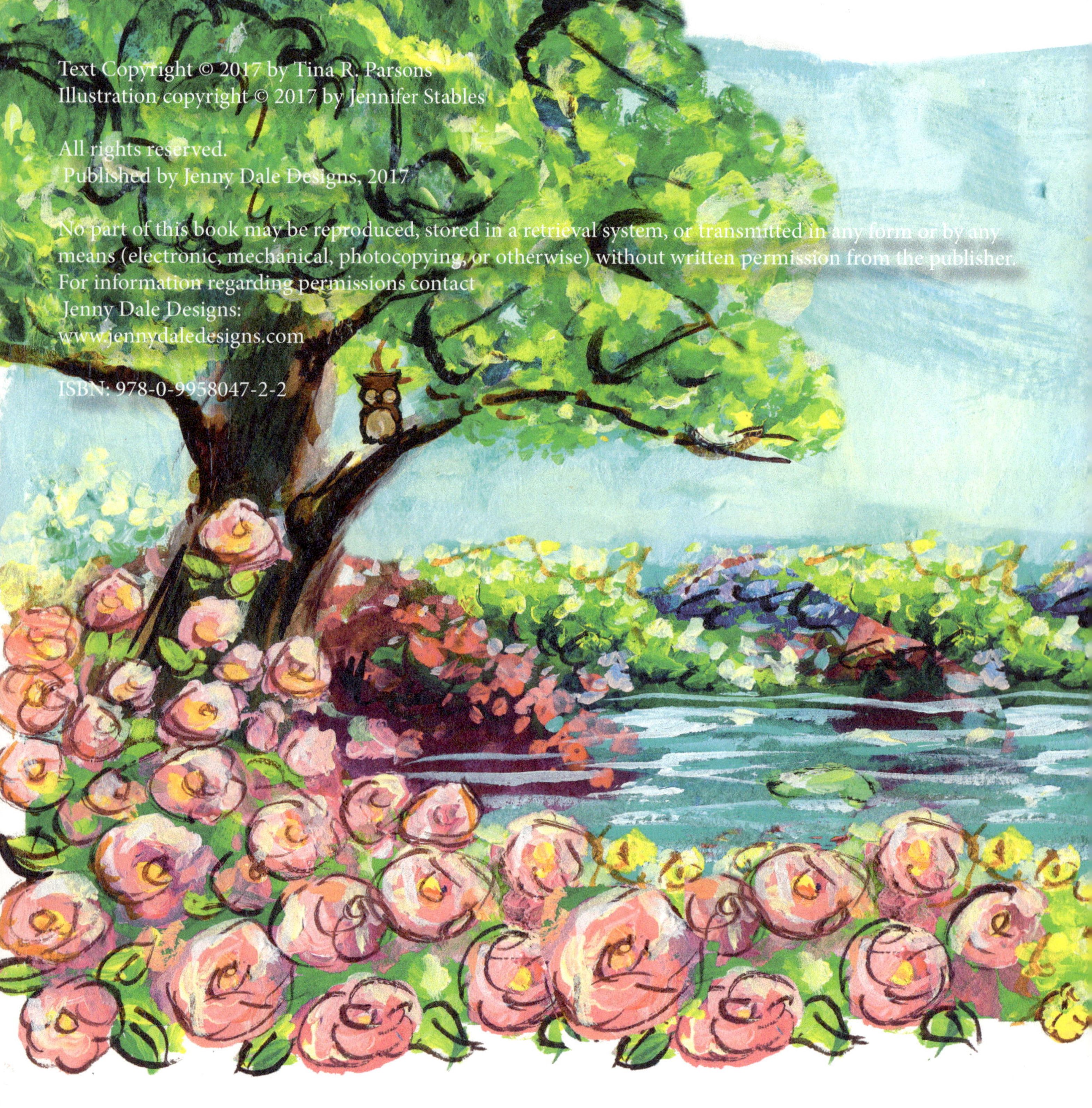

Published by Jenny Dale Designs, 2017

ISBN: 978-0-9958047-2-2

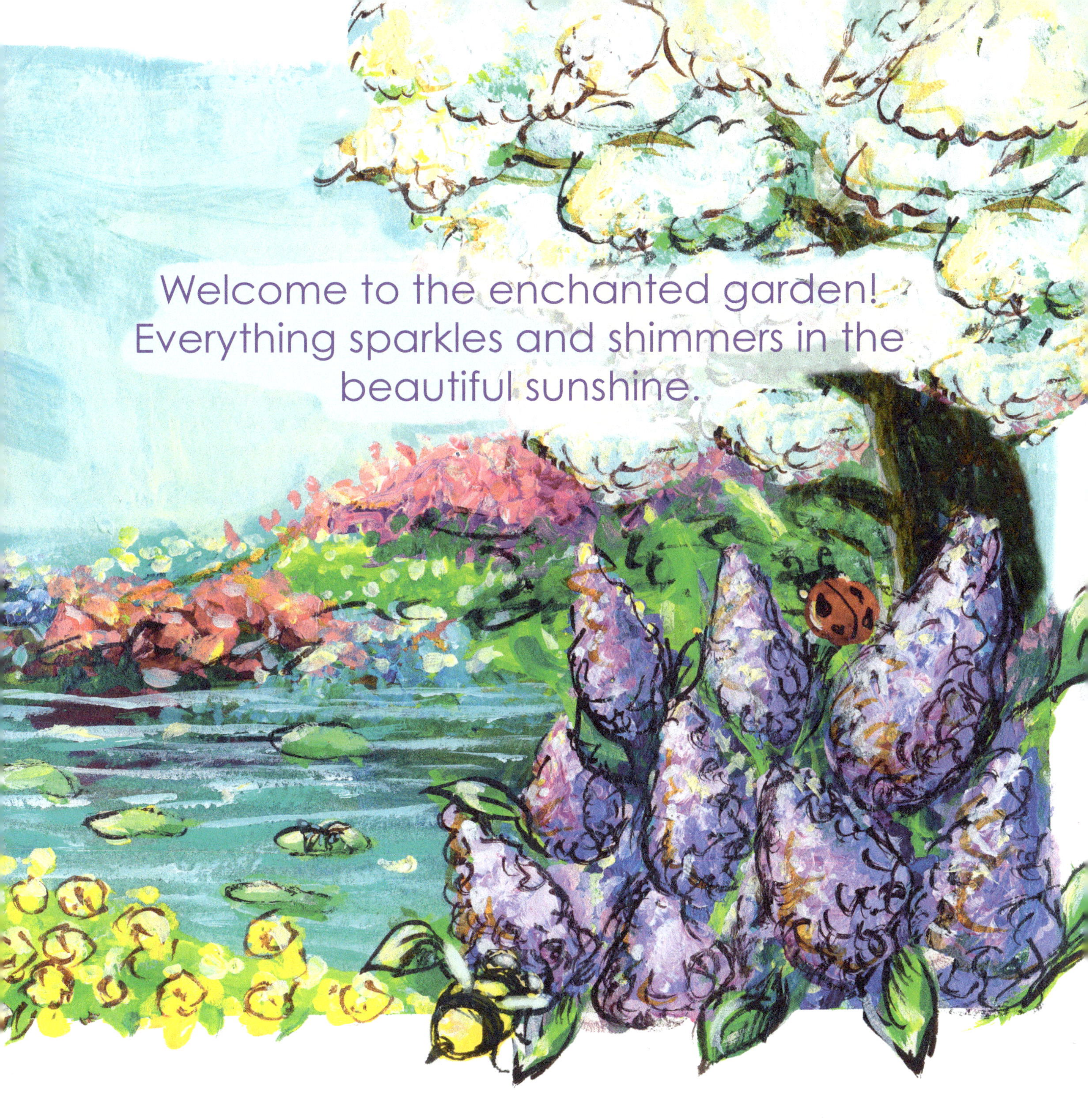

Welcome to the enchanted garden! Everything sparkles and shimmers in the beautiful sunshine.

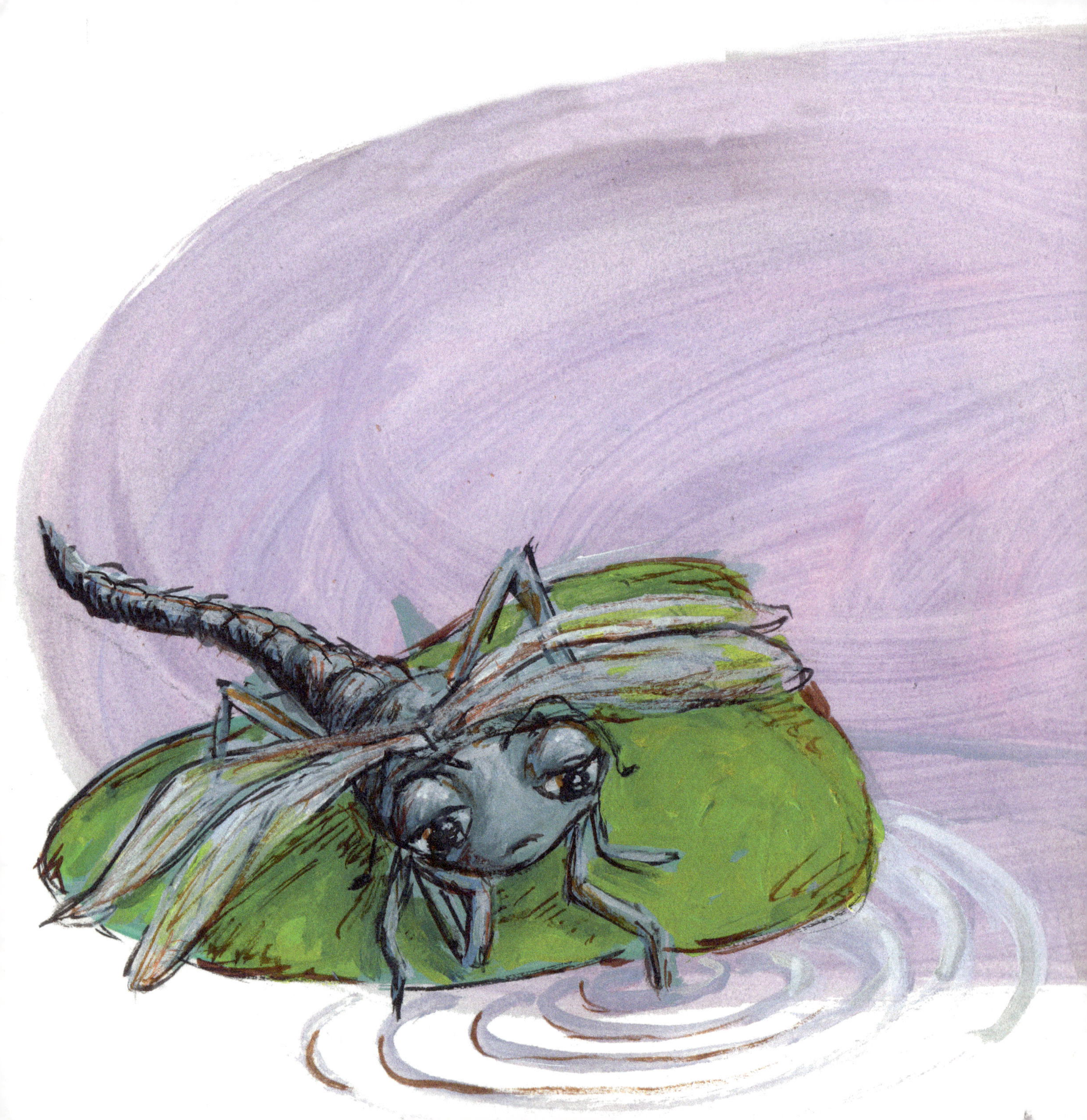

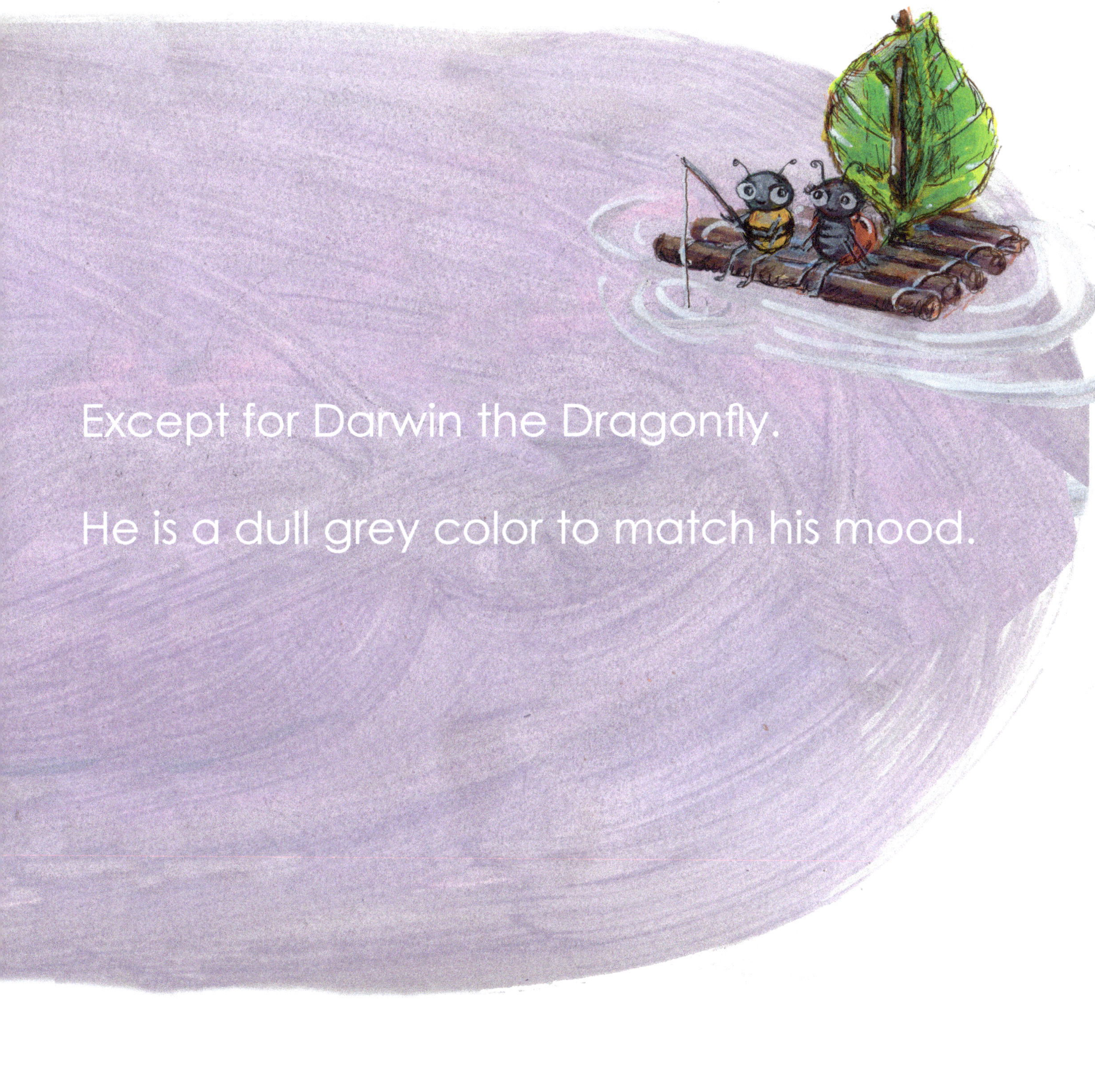

Except for Darwin the Dragonfly.

He is a dull grey color to match his mood.

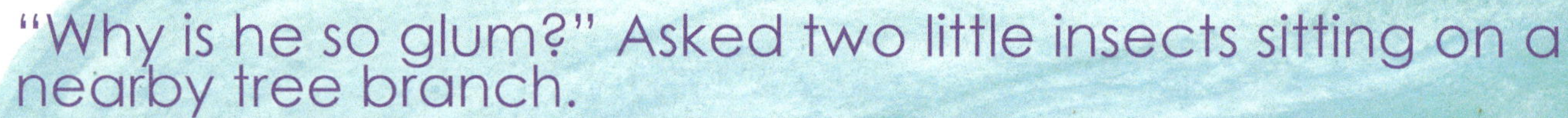

"Why is he so glum?" Asked two little insects sitting on a nearby tree branch.

A wise owl perched high in the tree answered, "Darwin does not know the secret of being mindful so he is often quite grumpy".

"Ohhhh", said the little insects in unison, "That's too bad".

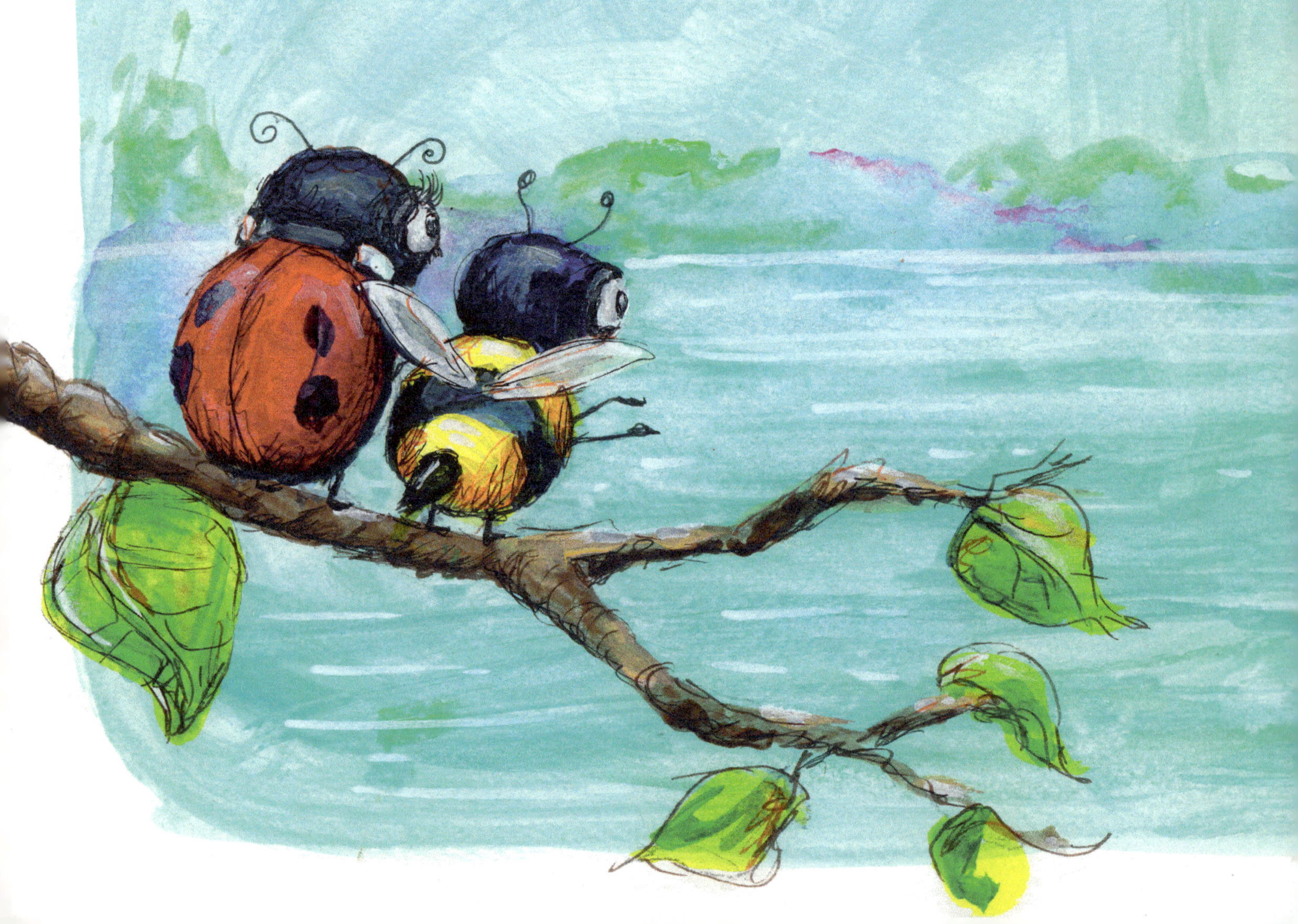

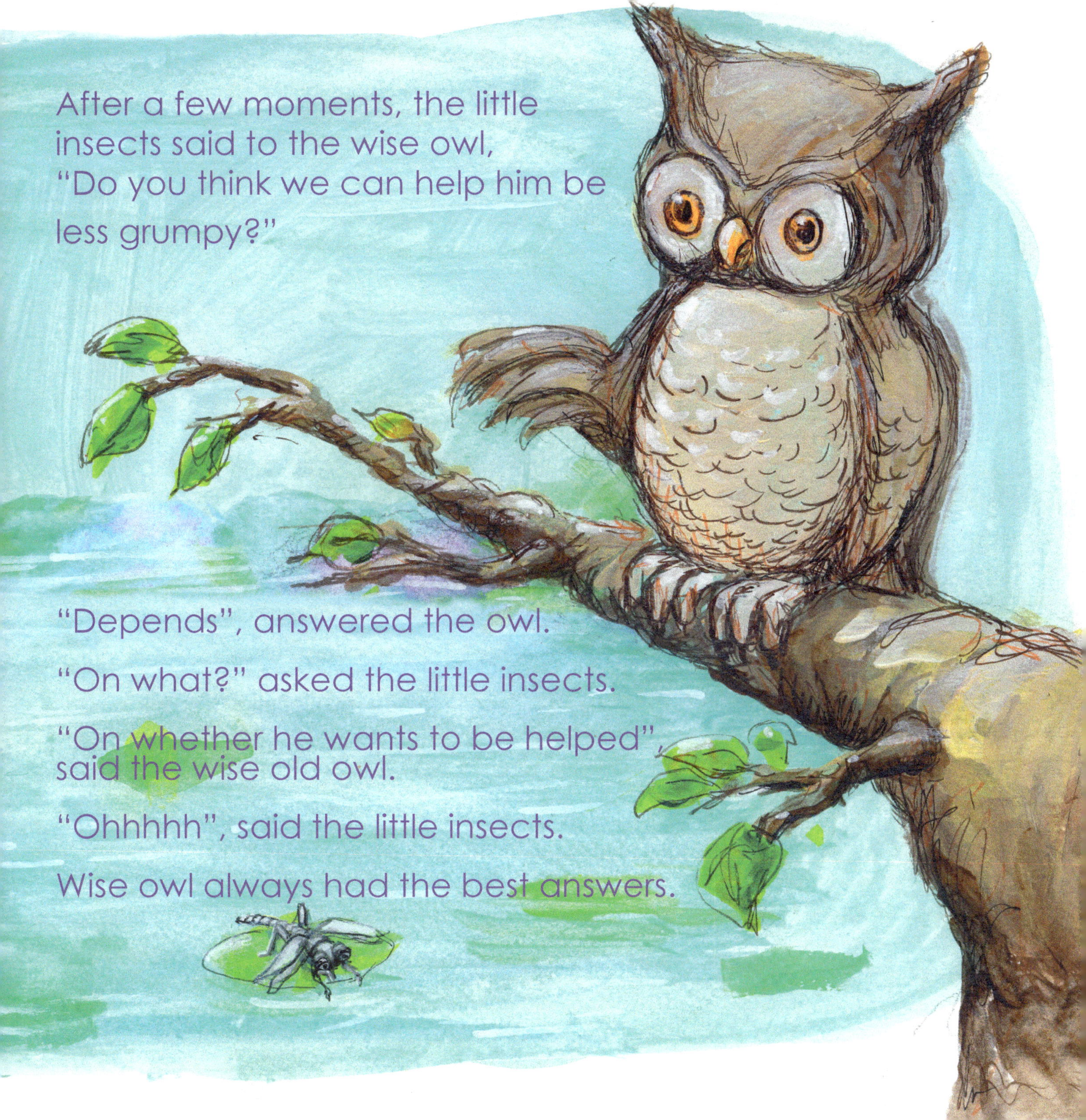

After a few moments, the little insects said to the wise owl, "Do you think we can help him be less grumpy?"

"Depends", answered the owl.

"On what?" asked the little insects.

"On whether he wants to be helped", said the wise old owl.

"Ohhhhh", said the little insects.

Wise owl always had the best answers.

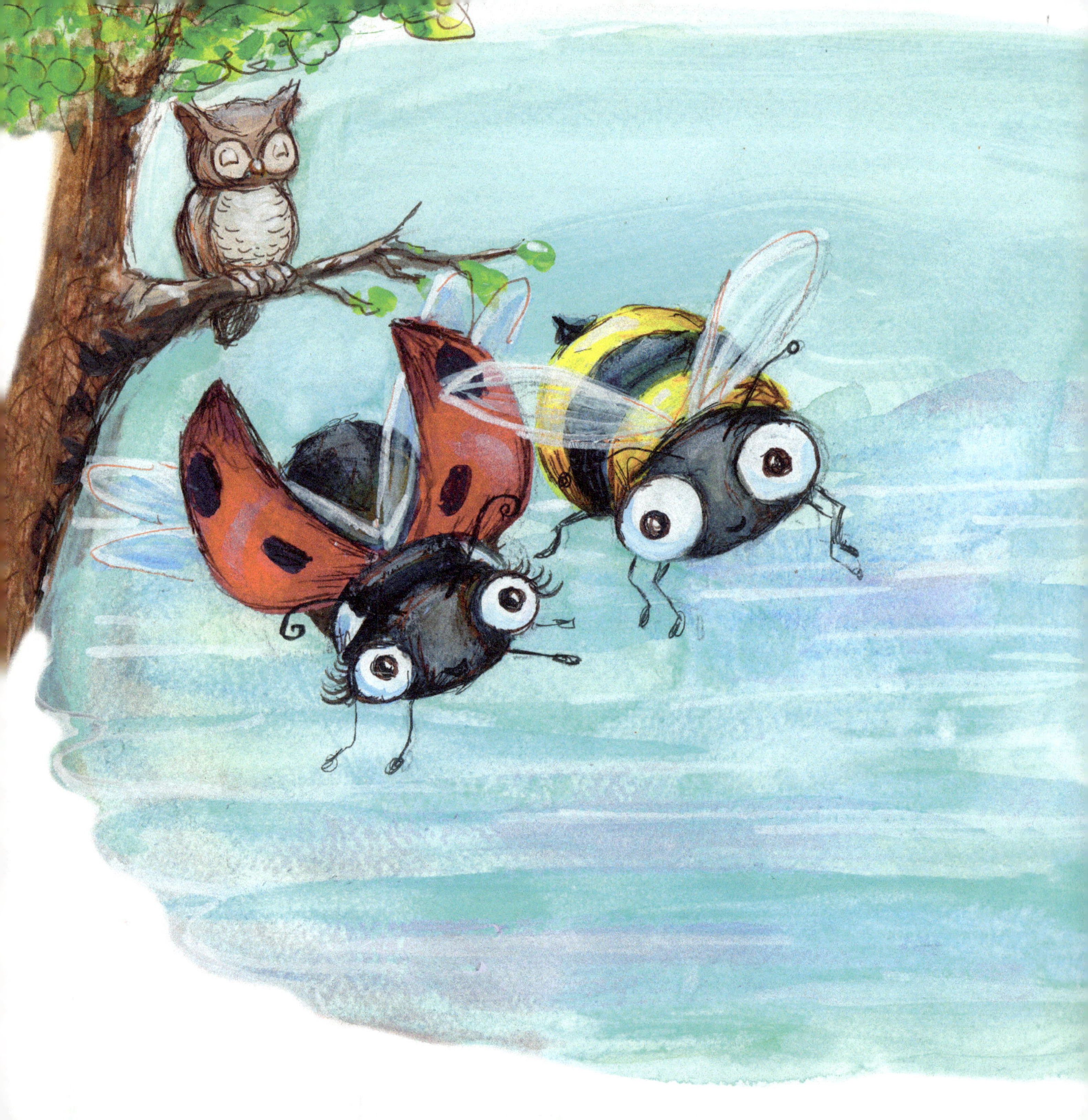

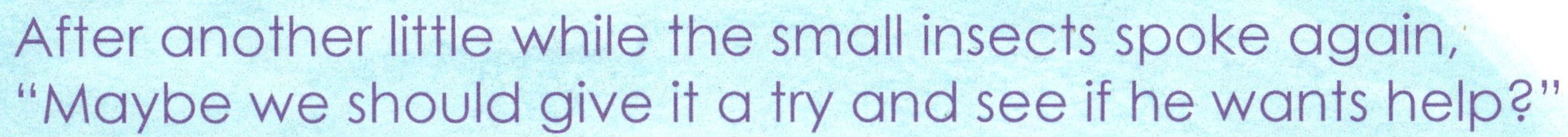

After another little while the small insects spoke again, "Maybe we should give it a try and see if he wants help?"

Wise owl just sat quietly with his eyes closed. Why did he always seem so calm, thought the little insects before deciding to fly down next to Darwin Dragonfly.

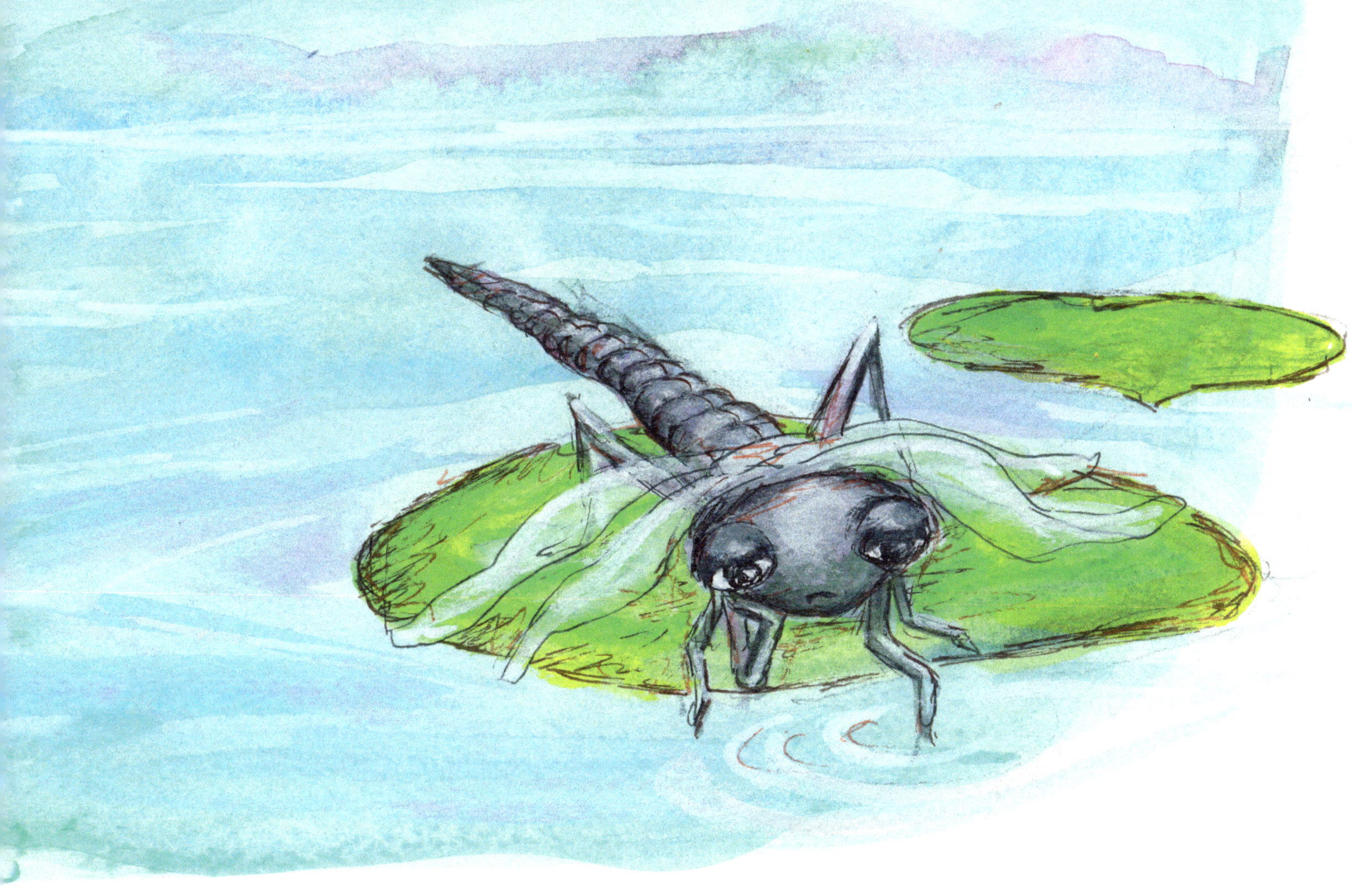

Darwin Dragonfly eyed them suspiciously.
"What do you want?" he asked grumpily.

"We want to help you", the tiny insects said in unison.

Darwin looked grumpier than ever and replied,
"Go away! Who says I need any help!"

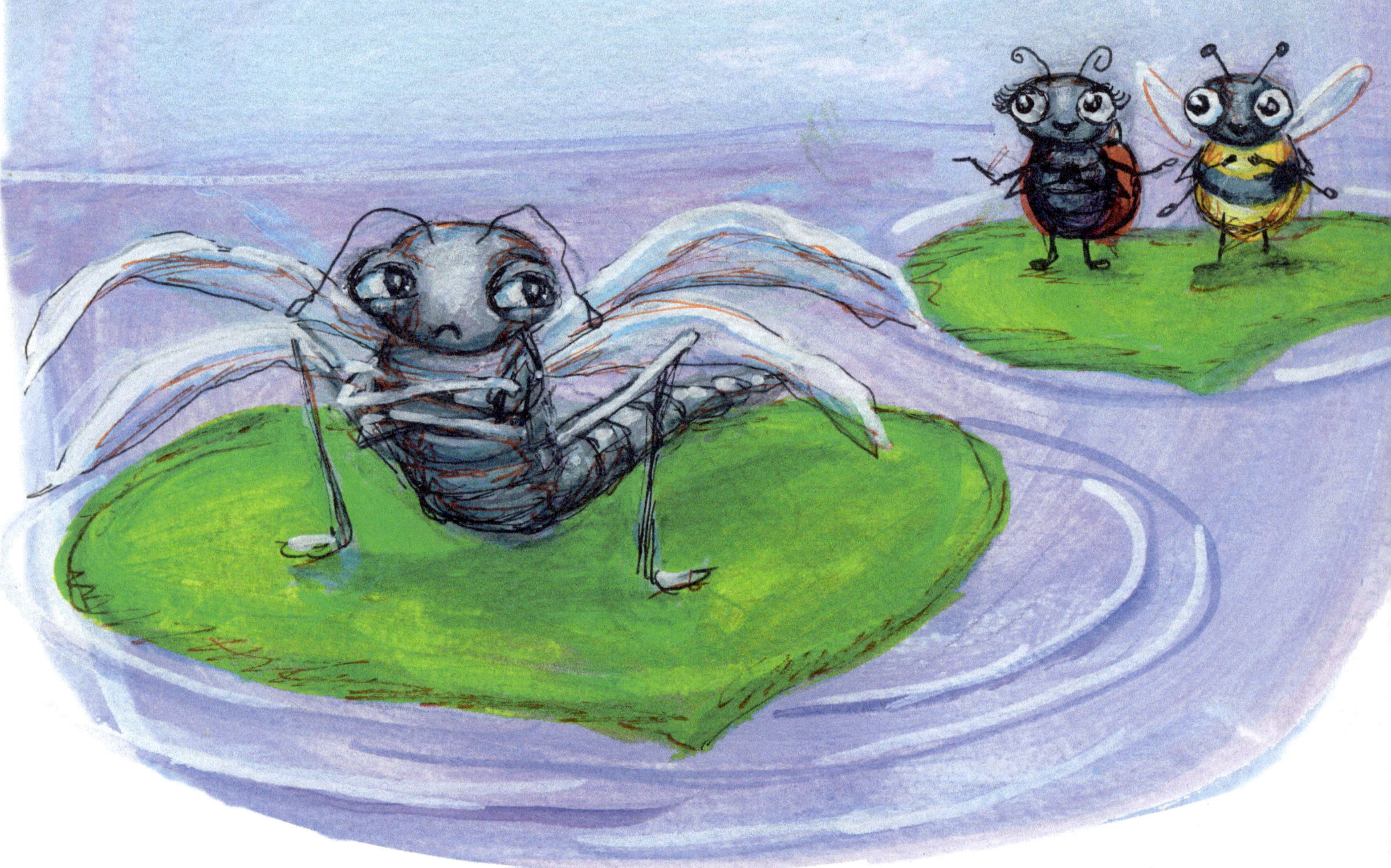

The small insects looked at each other in surprise and then back at Darwin. They quietly flew away leaving Darwin all alone.

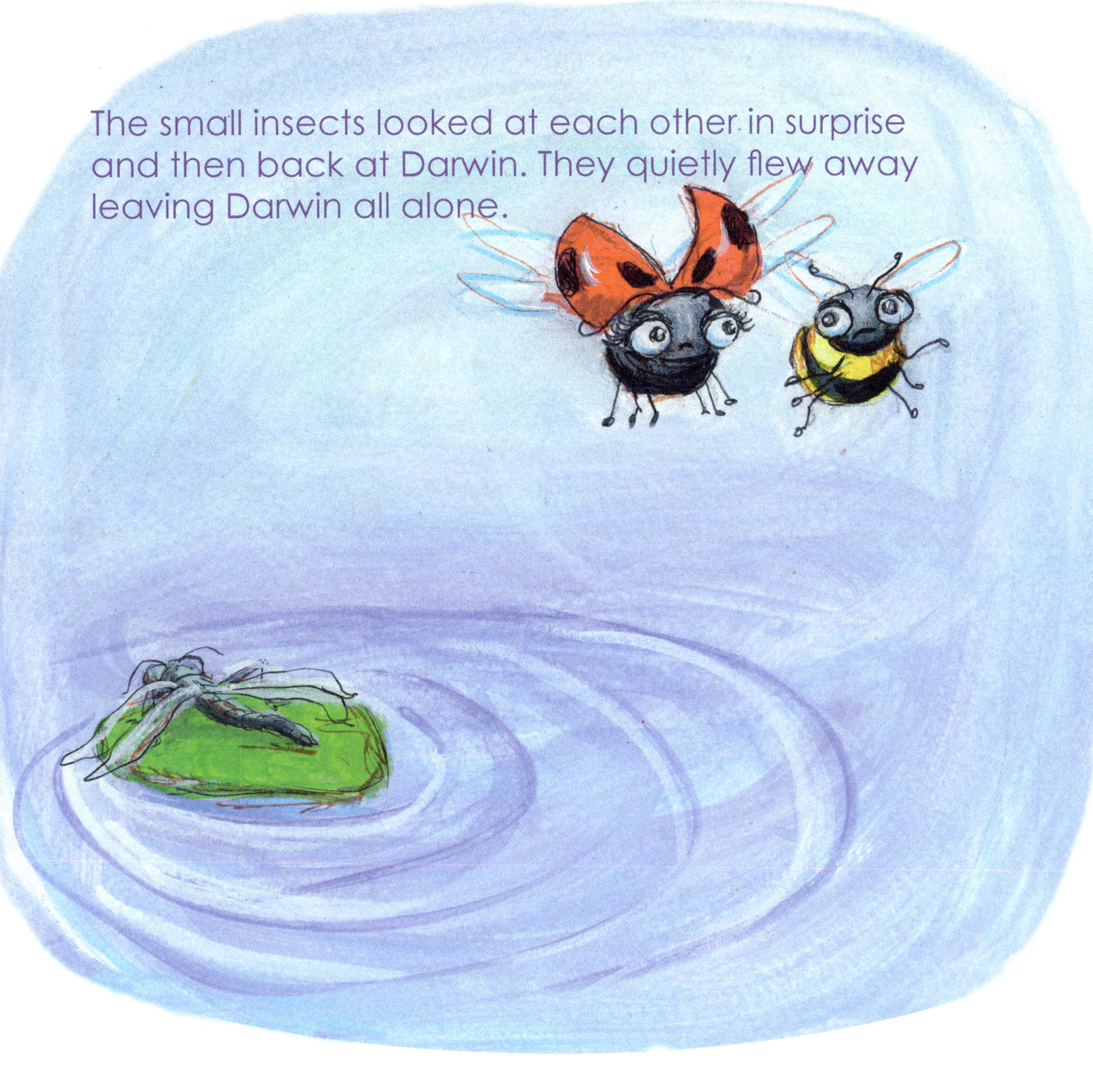

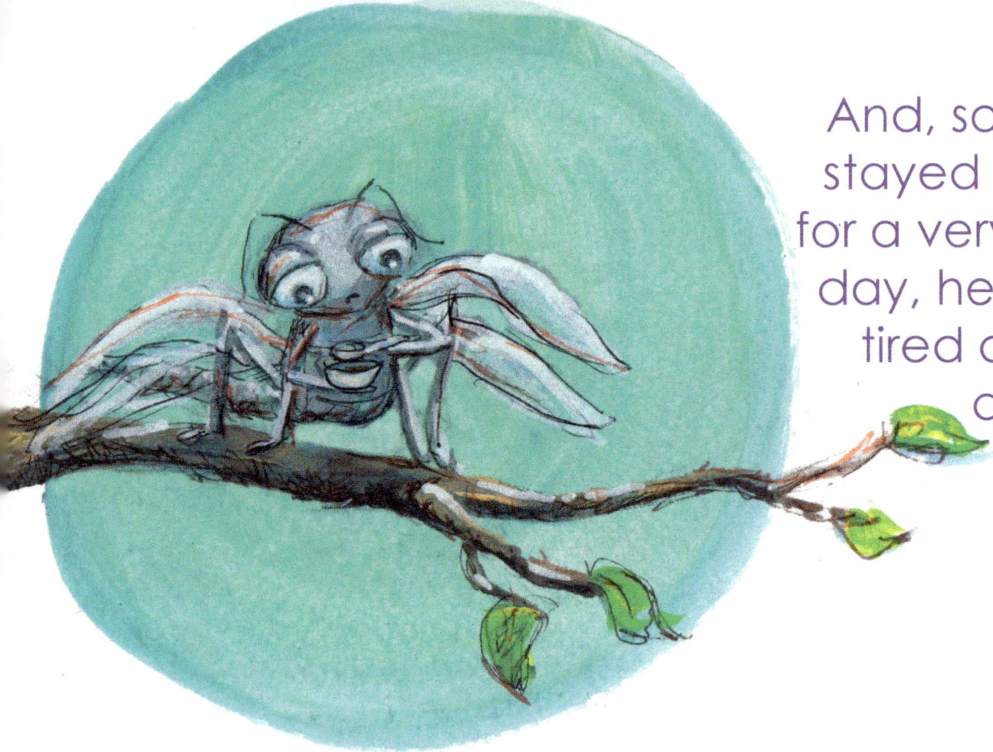

And, so it was that Darwin stayed grumpy and alone for a very long time until one day, he suddenly became tired of being grumpy and alone all the time.

He decided to try to find the small insects who had tried to be kind to him so long ago.

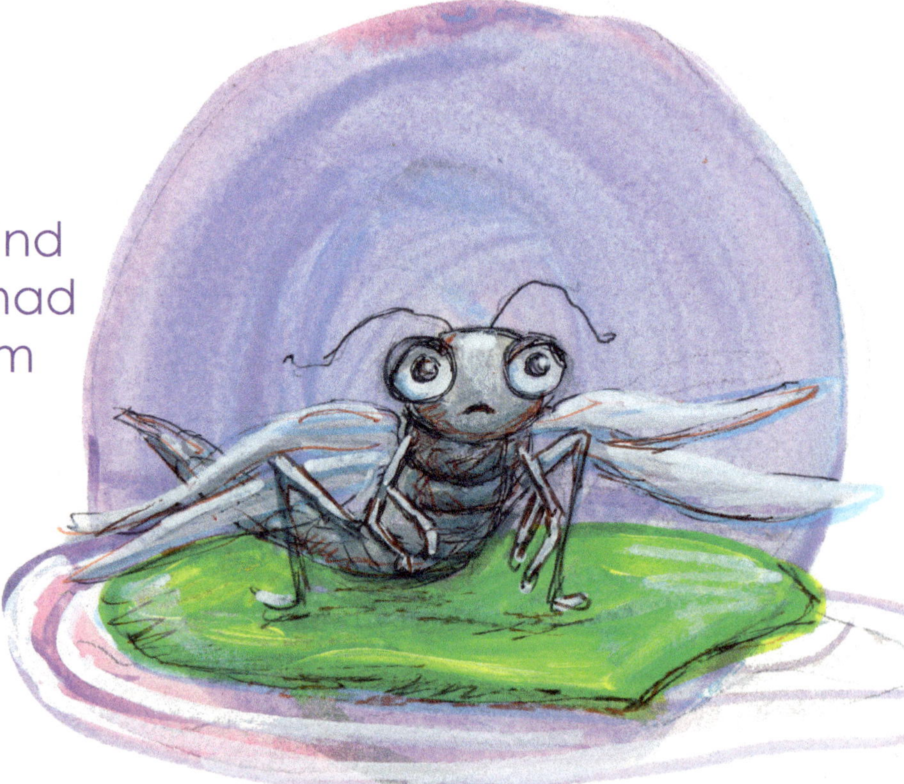

After many hours of searching, Darwin found them sitting on a tree branch enjoying the sun. Darwin cleared his voice and said, “Ahem, can you help me now?”

The little insects looked at each other in surprise and then back at Darwin. “Of course!” they said. And so they all set off to find wise owl who was, as usual sitting peacefully in the highest branches of a tree.

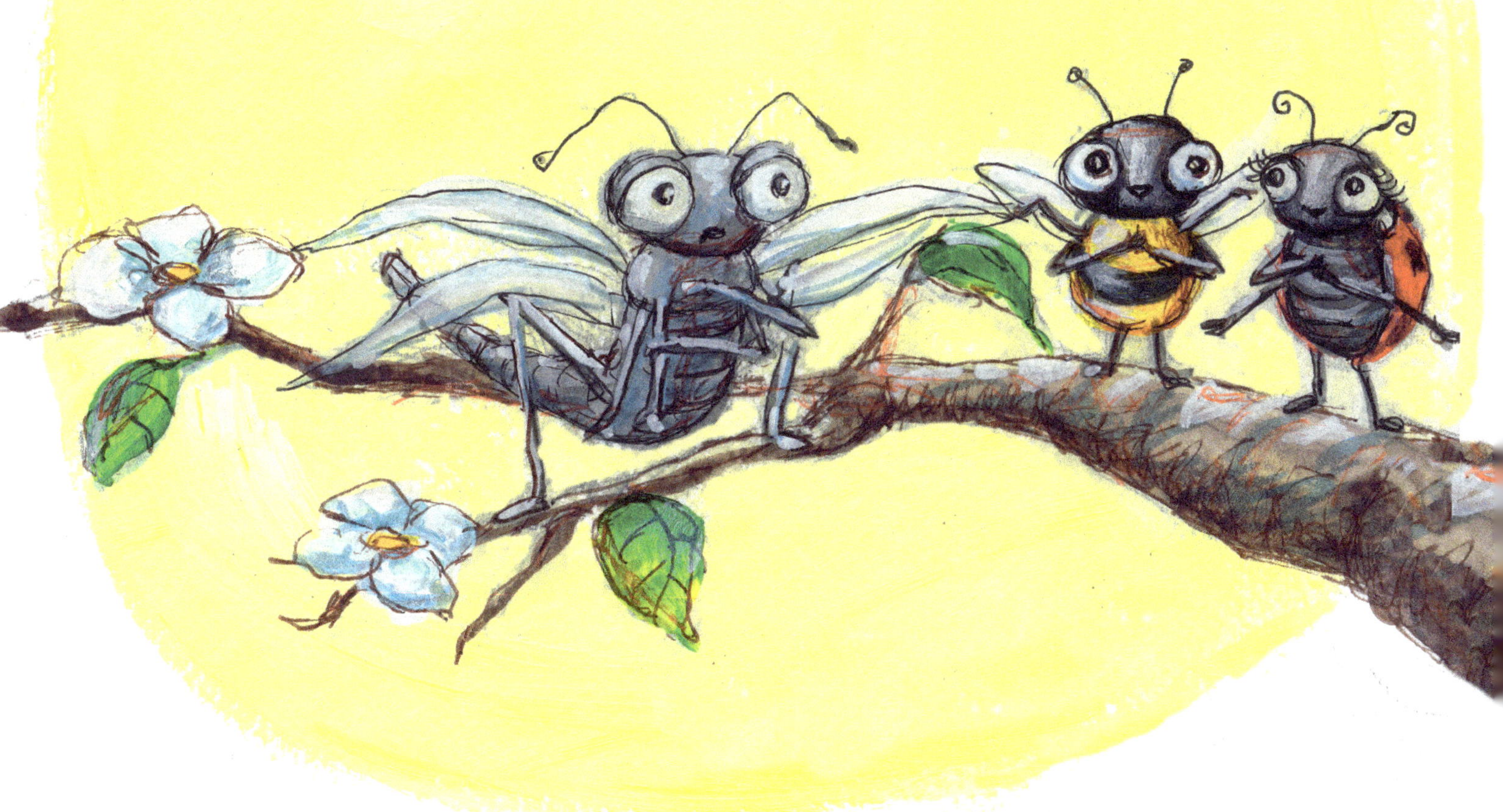

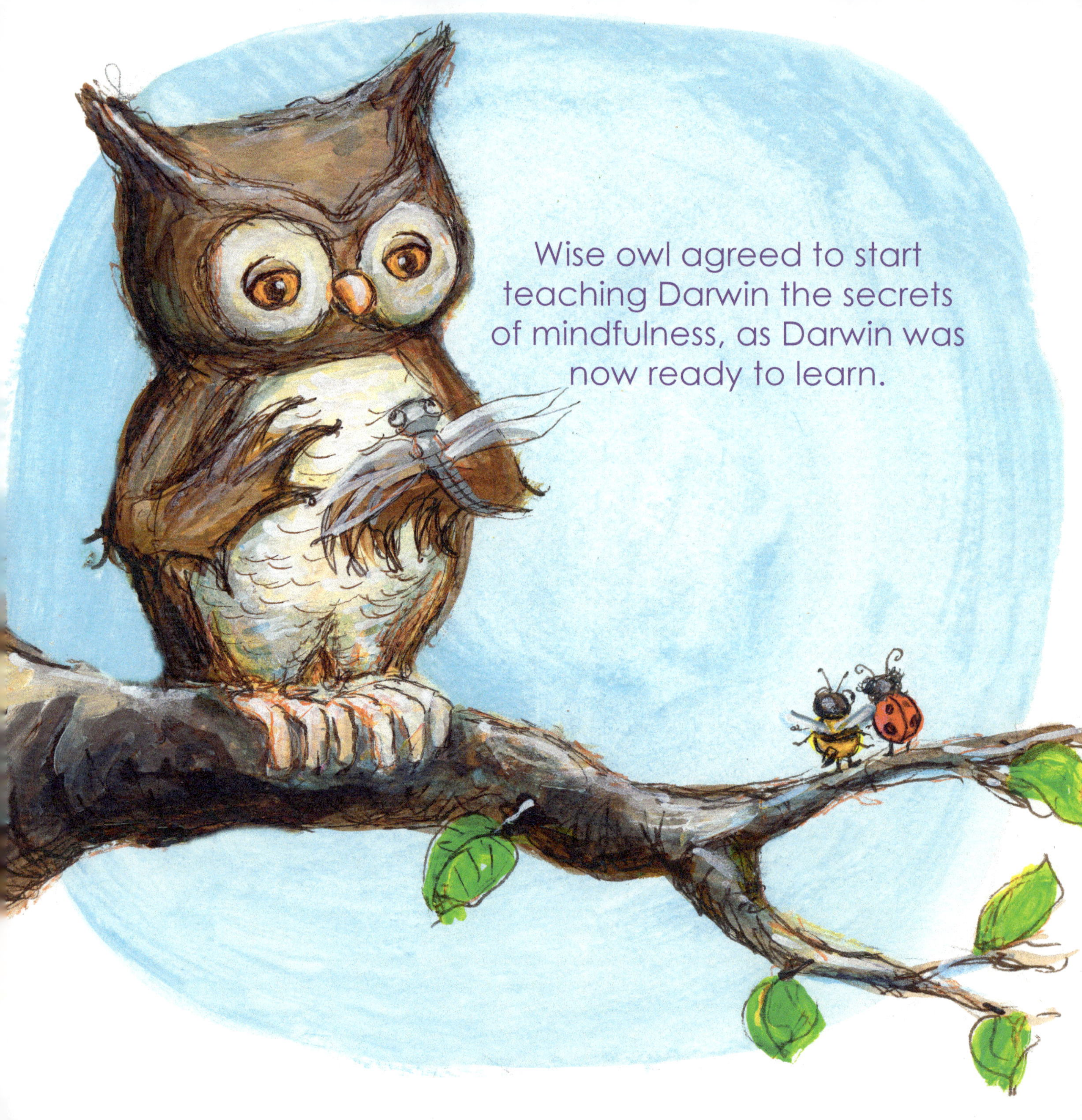

Wise owl agreed to start teaching Darwin the secrets of mindfulness, as Darwin was now ready to learn.

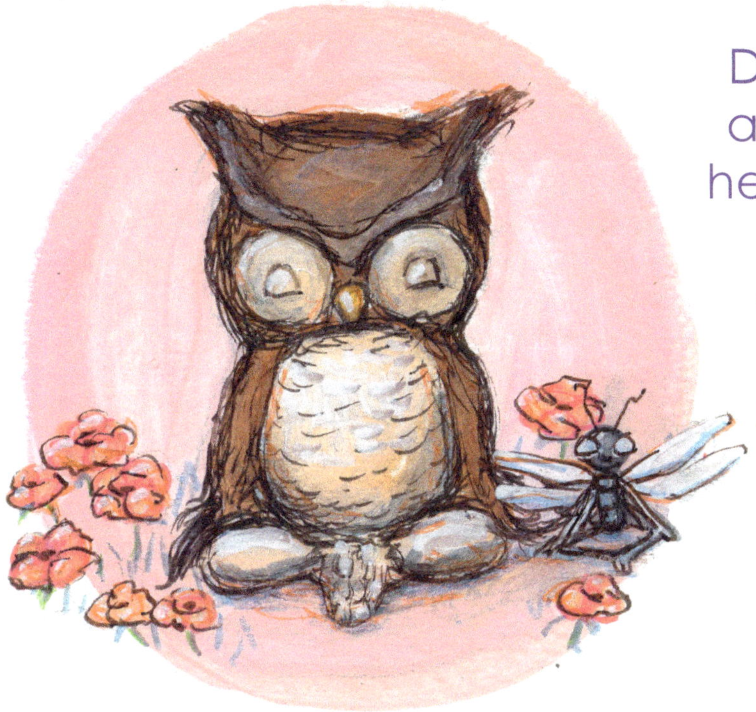

Darwin was a good student and he practiced daily until he was able to show wise owl and all the insects of the enchanted forest that he understood the secrets of living mindfully.

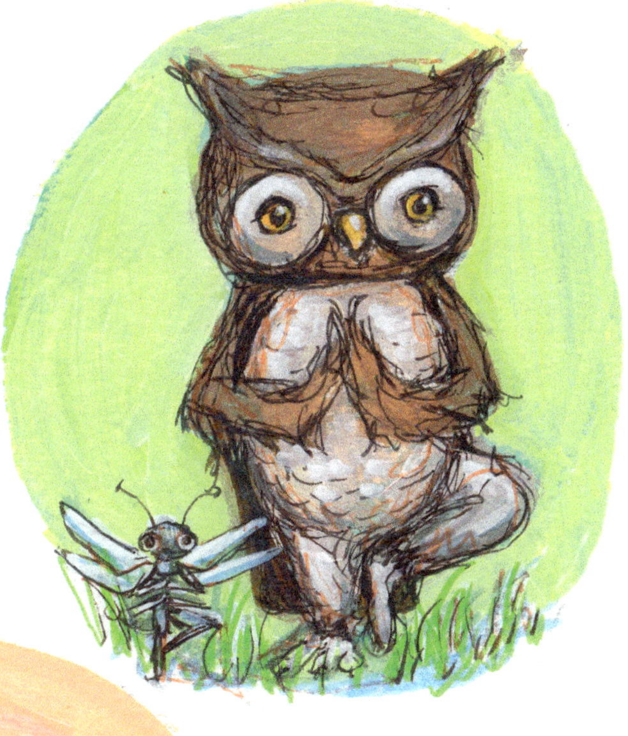

And how do they know that Darwin has changed?

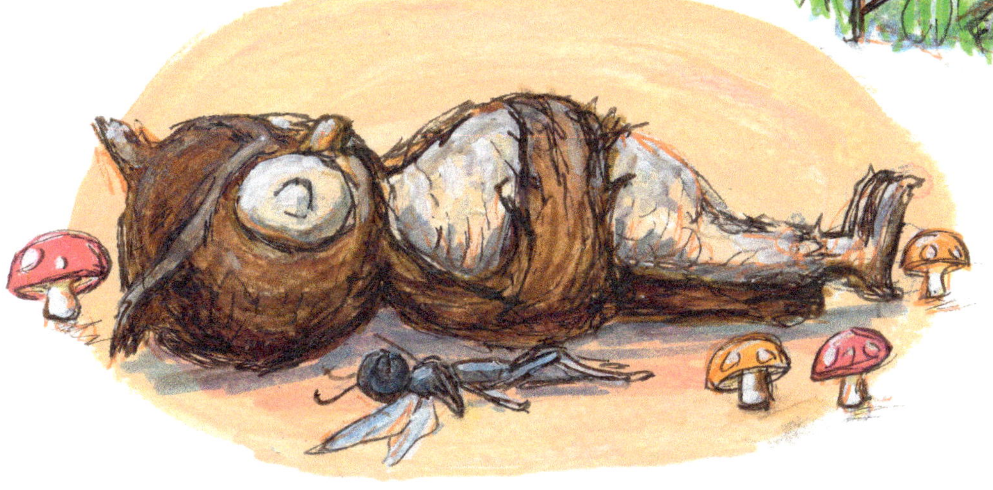

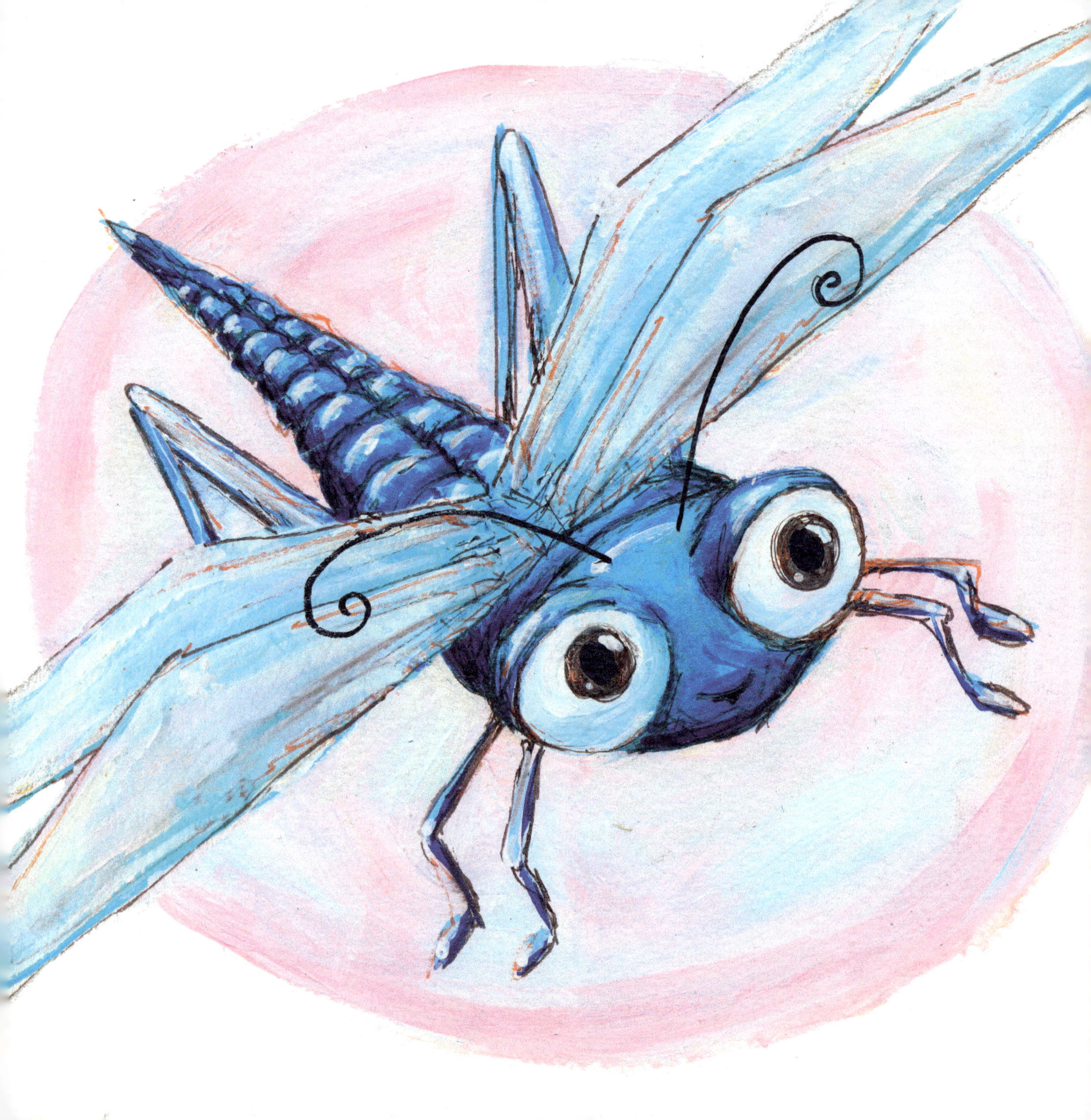

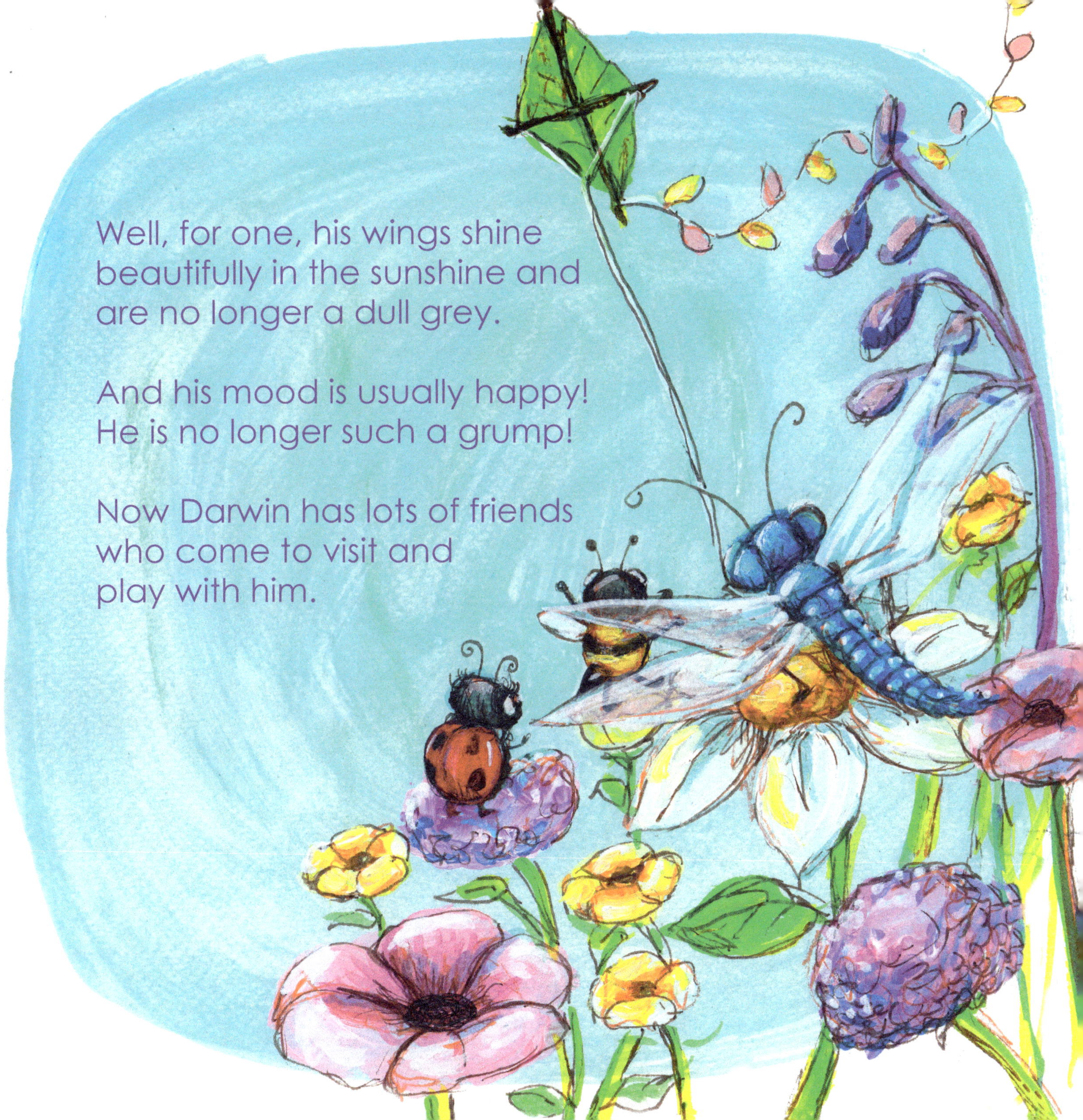

Well, for one, his wings shine beautifully in the sunshine and are no longer a dull grey.

And his mood is usually happy! He is no longer such a grump!

Now Darwin has lots of friends who come to visit and play with him.

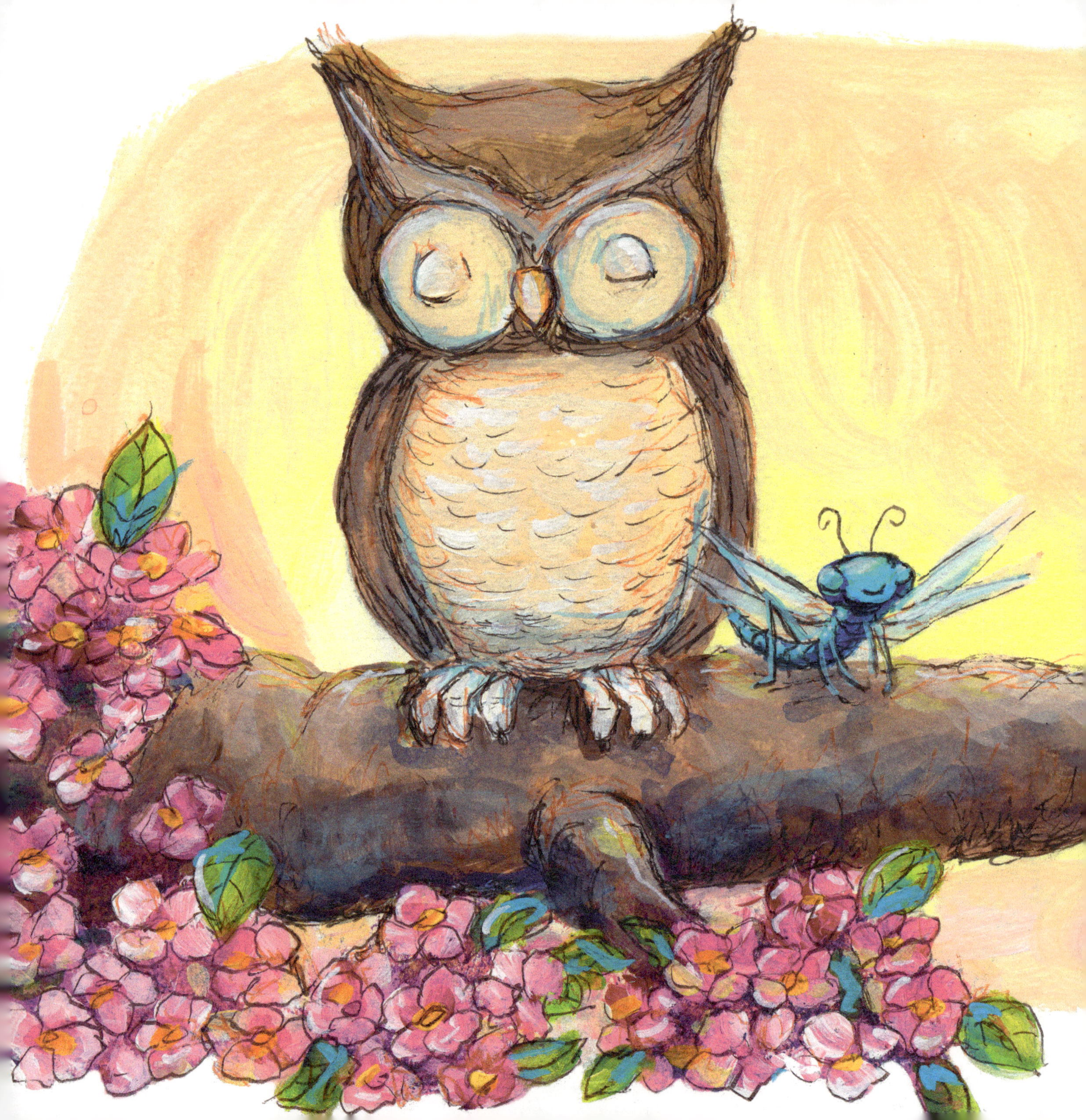

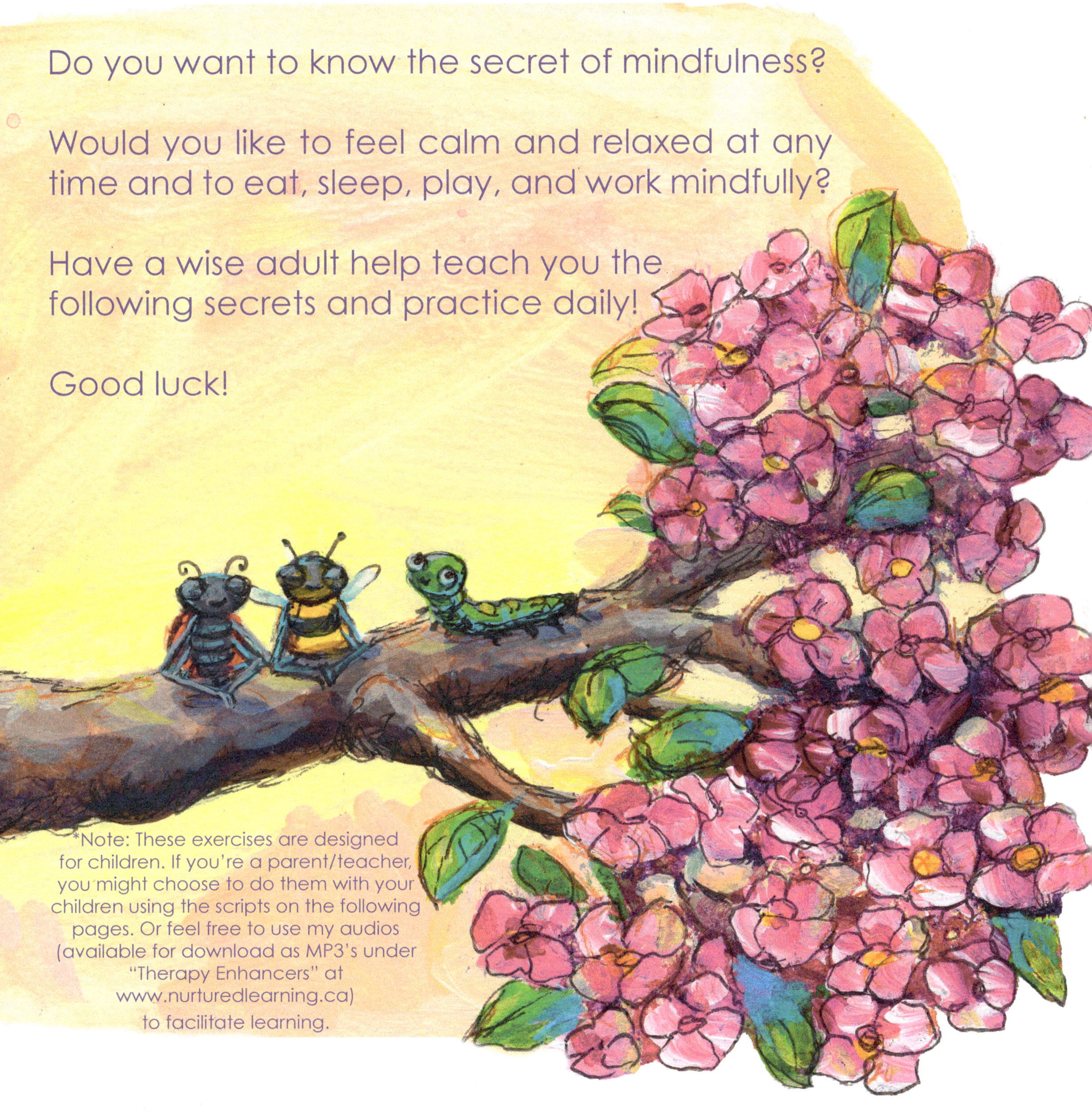

Do you want to know the secret of mindfulness?

Would you like to feel calm and relaxed at any time and to eat, sleep, play, and work mindfully?

Have a wise adult help teach you the following secrets and practice daily!

Good luck!

*Note: These exercises are designed for children. If you're a parent/teacher, you might choose to do them with your children using the scripts on the following pages. Or feel free to use my audios (available for download as MP3's under "Therapy Enhancers" at www.nurturedlearning.ca) to facilitate learning.

DEEP BREATHING

Note: We will now focus on how to correctly deep breathe. It is so important and essential. Most people are not even aware that they shallow breathe most of the time. They rush so quickly from one thing to another, even their breathing is rushed! You could also call this "big breathing" versus "small breathing". We will not advance to progressively relaxing muscles, body scan or noticing thoughts until we can deep breathe or "big breathe" properly. We should try to practice this every day for a few minutes throughout the day until we can naturally "go to our deep breath" when we are feeling stressed, tired or overwhelmed. If sitting, sit up nice and straight in a chair with the shoulders pulled "down and away from the ears" and the shoulder blades pulled gently together so that there is expansion through the chest and therefore easier to deep breathe. No slouching!

Script: Good, now let's begin. Sit or lie comfortably and close your eyes. Now, take one deep breath in through your nose. You should be able to count to at least three in your head while you are inhaling. Hold for one-two seconds before gently blowing all the air out through your nose or mouth (whichever is most comfortable for you). This should also take at least three seconds.

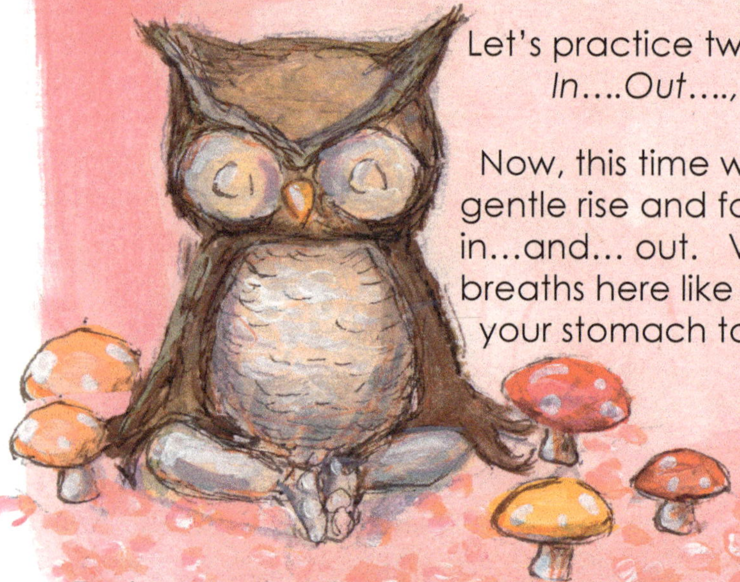

Let's practice two to three deep breaths here together.
In….Out…., In….Out….In….Out. Very good.

Now, this time while you are deep breathing, notice the gentle rise and fall of your stomach as you deeply breathe in…and… out. Very Good. Let's practice two-three deep breaths here like this. You may want to place your hand on your stomach to feel the gentle rise and fall as you breathe.
Very Good.

Try to practice like this each morning, at lunch and again at night before bed.

PROGRESSIVE MUSCLE RELAXATION

Script: Sit up nice and straight with your hands resting on your lap or lie down on your back. Get yourself into a comfortable position and close your eyes. Take three deep breaths. Pay attention to how calming this feels. Notice your stomach gently rising and falling as you deeply inhale and exhale. If you'd like, you can place your hand on your stomach and feel it moving in and out with each deep breath.

Now starting at your feet, spread your toes and relax the muscles in your feet. From the feet move slowly up to your legs. Relax the muscles in your lower legs and upper legs. Keep deep breathing!

Now spread and relax your fingers and the muscles in your hands. Notice your arms. Start to relax the muscles in your lower arms and upper arms. Now, relax your stomach, let it push out a bit. Relax your chest, pull your shoulders down and away from your ears, relax your back. Notice your head feels heavy.

Start to relax the muscles of the face, let your cheeks feel like they are sliding down your face. Soften your eyes and unclench your jaw. Notice that your whole body feels completely relaxed.

Continue deep breathing!

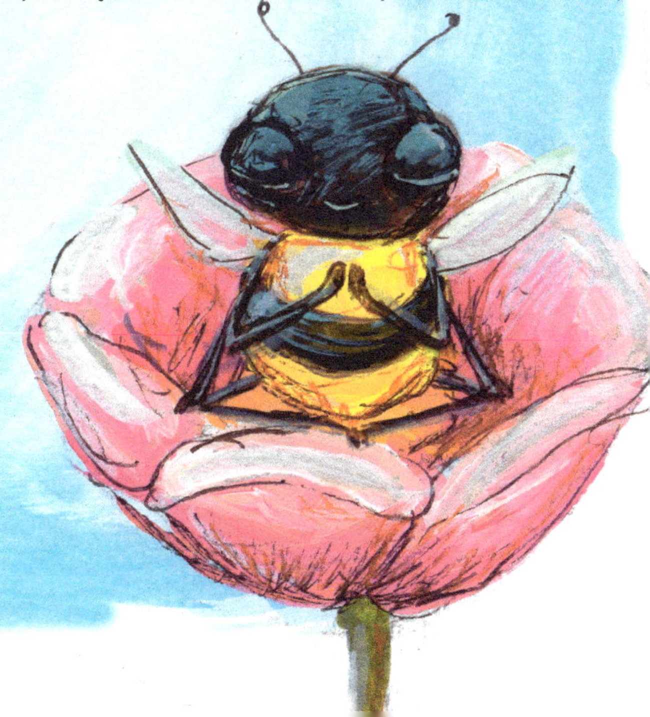

BODY SCAN

Script: Now, starting at the top of your head. Gently scan or become aware of each part of your body from the top of your head to the tips of your toes. Notice if there is any tension/discomfort in each area and if you find any, breathe deeply into those areas and see if you can relax your body even more.

NOTICING THOUGHTS

Script: Now, bring your attention to your mind. Just notice any thoughts that pop up in your mind without judgement. Simply observe each thought and watch it go by, like beautiful white clouds in a blue sky. Notice if your mind likes to spend most of it's time thinking about the past, the present or the future. You may also wish to notice if your thoughts are mostly positive, negative or neutral (neither positive nor negative).

Again, just observe without judgement. The practice of becoming aware of the content of your thoughts is an important one. If you practice like this every day, you will likely feel more peaceful, calm, and focused.

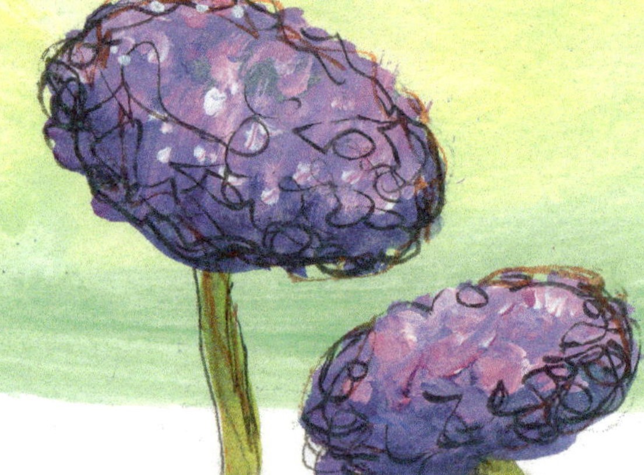

Now, for these last few minutes, let yourself be still.
There's nothing you need to do, nowhere you need to go.
If your mind gets busy, gently bring your attention back to your deep breathing again. If you feel that it's hard to focus, that's alright. Gently practice coming back again and again to how your stomach rises and falls with each deep breath.
You may even say in your mind, "breathing in....breathing out".
Do this until you feel calm.
Then, open your eyes and sit or lie for a few more moments to let your eyes adjust to the light and colors of the room.
Good job.

AHHH, NOW DOESN'T THAT FEEL BETTER?

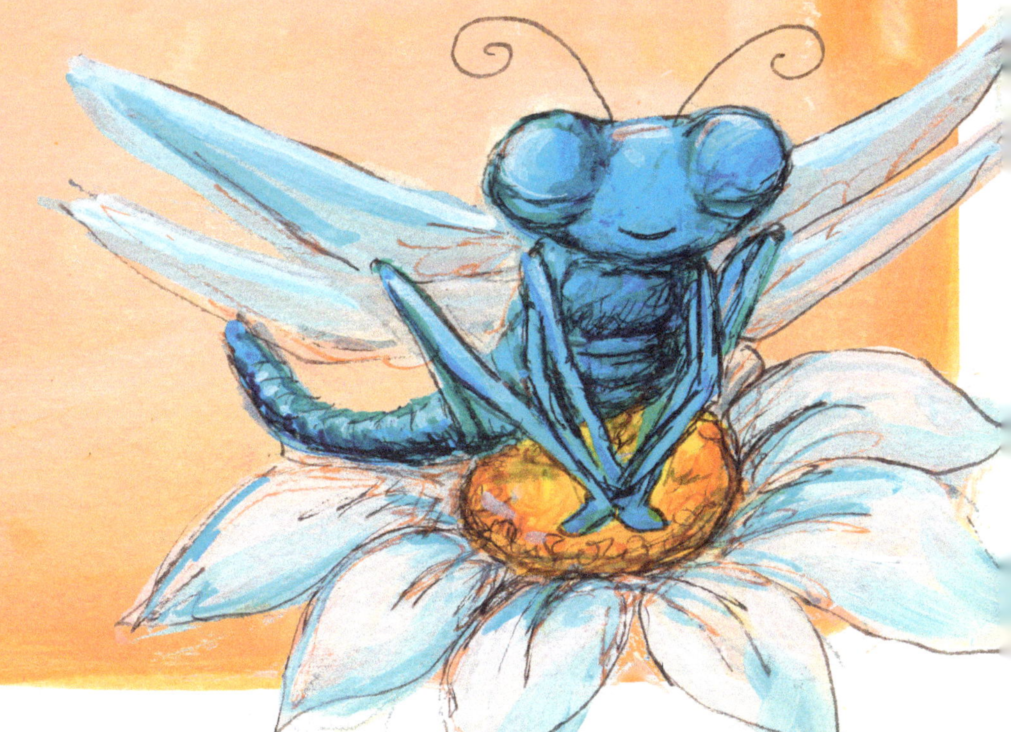

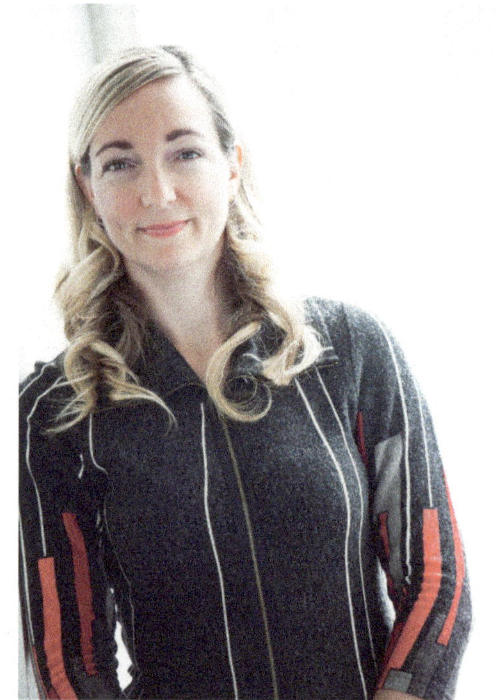

ABOUT THE AUTHOR

Tina R. Parsons is a Registered Psychologist from Calgary, Alberta, Canada who believes in the mind-body connection. She is also a certified fitness instructor and yoga instructor. She has a private practice (**www.nurturedlearning.ca**) where she works with children, adolescents and adults who are interested in developing their own mindfulness practice. She is married with two children.

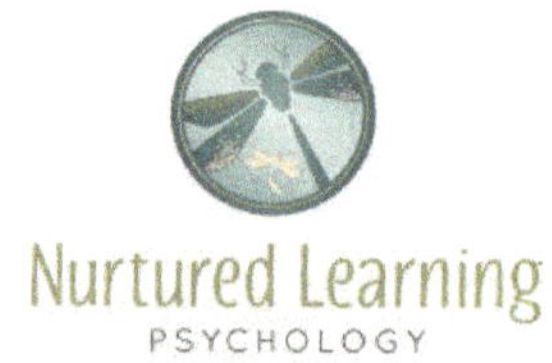

ABOUT THE ILLUSTRATOR

Jennifer Dale Stables, B.F.A., B.Ed., is an artist and educator living in Okotoks, Alberta, Canada. A former classroom teacher, Jennifer has dedicated her artistic endeavors to creating artwork and illustrations for children. Through her business, Jenny Dale Designs, she creates whimsical artwork and writes poetry to accompany each one of her lovable creations. She is married with two children.

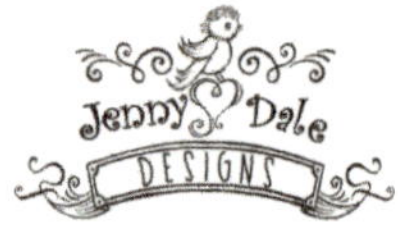

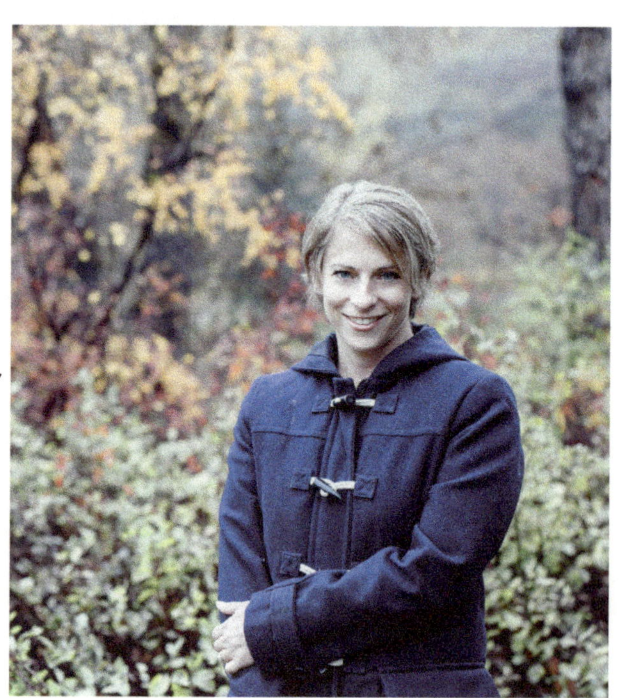

CPSIA information can be obtained
at www.ICGtesting.com
Printed in the USA
LVHW07s2315201018
594210LV00003B/3/P